POCKET SERIES FOR MRCP PART 2

BOOK 1

Cardiology & Respiratory Medicine

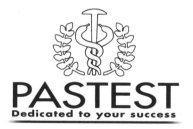

PASTEST
Dedicated to your success

POCKET SERIES FOR MRCP PART 2

BOOK 1
Cardiology & Respiratory Medicine

Edited by Richard L. Hawkins MBBS FRCS

Cardiology:
David Smith MB ChB MRCP
St Thomas' Hospital, London

Respiratory Medicine:
Stefan Lozewicz MD MRCP
John Moore-Gillon MA MD MRCP
St Bartholomew's Hospital, London

© 1990 PASTEST
Egerton Court, Parkgate Estate, Knutsford
Cheshire WA16 8DX
Tel: 01565 752000

First printed in 1990
Reprinted 1995
Reprinted 1999

A catalogue reference for this title is available from the British Library.

ISBN 0 906896 37 1

Text prepared by Turner Associates, Knutsford, Cheshire
Phototypeset by Speedset Ltd, Ellesmere Port, Cheshire
Printed in Great Britain by The Cromwell Press, Trowbridge, Wilts

CONTENTS

BIBLIOGRAPHY

CARDIOLOGY
Cardiology Pocket Consultant. R. H. Swanton. 3rd ed.
1994 Blackwell Scientific.

RESPIRATORY MEDICINE
Respiratory Diseases. J. Crofton and A. Douglas. 4th ed.
1989 Blackwell Scientific.
The Heart. W. Hurst. 6th ed. 1985 McGraw Hill.
Oxford Textbook of Medicine. 3rd ed. 1995 Oxford University Press.

INTRODUCTION

The MRCP Part 2 Examination is a test of competent clinical practice as opposed to the theoretical knowledge required for Part 1. The examiners want to be reassured that the candidate is professional in his or her approach and manner, accomplished in technique, safe in practice and honest in ignorance. There is no doubt that efficient, systematic preparation for the Part 2 can make all the difference between passing and failing the examination. Familiarity with the type of questions being set, together with a knowledge of how best to present the answers and how they are marked by the examiners, will all help candidates to do their best in the examination.

Each of these three PasTest pocket books contain sample case histories and data interpretations carefully written and edited by doctors involved in the teaching and preparation of candidates for the MRCP examination. The case material, data and questions presented have all been chosen for their similarity to those experienced in recent official examinations:

Book 1: Cardiology and Respiratory Medicine
Book 2: Gastroenterology, Endocrinology and Renal Medicine
Book 3: Haematology, Rheumatology and Neurology.

The best way to use these books is to work through each question in a methodical manner keeping to the time limits set by the Royal College. This will give useful practice in coming to quick decisions about the answers, which can then be looked up, corrected and thought about in a more leisurely manner.

By working through these books and studying the correct answers and teaching notes, a candidate will be able to pinpoint specific topics and subject areas where further reading and study would be beneficial before the examination. **Please note that the correct answers given in these books are not presented in a simple list as required by the College on examination day, but are incorporated within the teaching notes.**

The written section of the examination consists of three question papers:

(a) Case Histories (four or more compulsory questions in 55 minutes.)
(b) Data Interpretation (ten compulsory questions in 45 minutes.)
(c) Projected Material (twenty compulsory questions in 40 minutes.)

The Royal College has published a booklet of 2 past MRCP Part 2 written examinations (general medicine and paediatrics) and all candidates would be wise to be familiar with these, in particular the simple answer format preferred.

Advice on How to Answer the Questions

The written part of the MRCP Part 2 examination has been designed to require minimal writing so that maximum time may be devoted by the candidate to thinking through the problems presented while, at the same time, it allows for objective marking by the examiners. This means that marks are awarded by the examiners in a predetermined manner. Specific answers are required and so candidates must listen carefully to the invigilator's instructions and understand exactly how to present their answers. Since specific answers are required, it is of no use to treat the questions as short answer questions in which you attempt to explain your thoughts to the examiner. Answers should be precise, yet complete, in their meaning. Vague answers score significantly lower marks.

Each question asks for a specific number of answers. Correct answers to a question will receive maximum marks but since there may be more than one possible correct answer, marks will be awarded on a scale according to their acceptibility. Where the 'best' answer is much better than the others, the difference in marking between the best and the other answers will be greater. Answers in excess of the number requested will be ignored. For example, if three diagnoses are given instead of two, only the first two will be marked, even if the third represents the best response. Space is given in the examination paper for each of your answers and it will be of considerable help to the examiners if you confine your answers to one per line.

All three papers in the written section are ascribed the same maximum number of marks. The final score for each candidate is the aggregate mark of all three papers. In order to pass, it is not necessary therefore to obtain a pass mark in each of the three papers, so long as the aggregate mark reaches the required pass mark.

Candidates who pass the written section are invited to attend for further examination in the clinical and oral sections. Those who marginally fail the written section may also proceed to the clinical and oral sections but, to succeed in the examination as a whole, have to obtain additional marks in these last two sections.

Candidates who have clearly failed the written section are deemed to have failed the examination as a whole and must resit the written section in order to proceed in the examination.

It is hoped that the material provided in these three pocket books will prove instrumental in the success of many Part 2 candidates.

CARDIOLOGY : CASE HISTORIES

1. A 32 year old mechanic is referred to you with a three-month history of severe breathlessness. He has been diagnosed as having a viral cardiomyopathy affecting the right ventricle and is now treated with diuretics and an angiotensin converting enzyme inhibitor. He was perfectly well until three months ago and served in the army five years previously.

   On examination he looked well. Pulse regular 80/min, BP 110/70 mm Hg. His jugular venous pressure was raised 4 cm with 'a' wave equal to 'v' wave. Auscultation revealed a wide split second heart sound and a systolic murmur, heard best at the left sternal border.

   The ECG showed right bundle branch block and a mean frontal QRS axis of 110°.

   Questions:

   1. What is the cause of his breathlessness?
   2. What abnormality would you see on the chest X-ray?
   3. What would be your investigation of choice and why?

2. A 17 year old male complains of rapid palpitations unrelated to exertion. Examination reveals mild central cyanosis, a regular pulse of 80/min, a raised venous pressure with a systolic wave, and a pansystolic murmur heard best at the left sternal edge which intensifies on inspiration. Hepatomegaly is also present.

   The ECG shows sinus rhythm, a PR interval of 0.10 seconds and a delta wave consistent with Wolff-Parkinson-White (W-P-W) syndrome type B.

   Questions:

   1. What is the diagnosis?
   2. What would be your next investigation?

Answers overleaf

1. 1. A secundum atrial septal defect. Congenital pulmonary stenosis is highly unlikely for three reasons. It produces a murmur that is likely to have been heard at the medical examination required to enter the armed forces, it causes right ventricular hypertrophy which gives rise to a dominant 'a' wave in the venous pressure, and the pulmonary component of the second heart sound tends to be soft or absent.

    2. Pulmonary plethora.

    3. Either cross-sectional echocardiography with colour flow doppler or cardiac catheterisation is required. The former has the advantage of being cheap, widely available and non-invasive but has three disadvantages: false negatives, difficulty in measuring the shunt and difficulty in adequately demonstrating associated abnormal venous drainage. Cardiac catheterisation, on the other hand, is not so widely available and is invasive, but has a low failure rate for finding the defect, gives definitive haemodynamic data and can and should be used to demonstrate normal systemic and pulmonary venous drainage.

2. 1. Ebstein's anomaly. This congenital abnormality is characterised by downward displacement of the tricuspid valve attachment. There is a broad spectrum of severity ranging from life threatening cases in infancy to chance findings at postmortem after a normal life span. The valve is often abnormal having hypoplastic, fused or perforated leaflets. Part of the right ventricle is 'atrialised' and the right ventricular stroke volume may be small. There is tricuspid regurgitation. A patent foramen ovale is common and right to left shunting through it accounts for arterial desaturation. Associated abnormalities of the conduction system often give rise to accessory bundles and W-P-W syndrome type B is a common finding. The large right atrium and W-P-W syndrome often cause supraventricular tachycardia so that palpitation is a frequent presenting complaint.

    2. Two-dimensional echocardiography. This clearly demonstrates the tricuspid displacement and the large 'atrialised' portion of the right ventricle.

3. A 42 year old woman is admitted to hospital following a collapse
and a fit in a restaurant. She gives a history of four previous
blackouts over the last 23 years, two of them followed by fits.
Each episode has been preceded by exercise or a meal.

On admission she is a well looking woman with no abnormal
neurological signs. Her pulse is 60/min, regular, with a slow upstroke
but a normal volume. Peripheral pulses are normal. On auscultation she has normal heart sounds with a loud ejection systolic
murmur heard throughout the praecordium and radiating to the
carotids.

The ECG shows sinus rhythm and left ventricular hypertrophy. The
echocardiogram is reported to show a normal aortic valve.

Questions:

1. What is the most likely diagnosis?
2. How would you confirm the diagnosis?
3. What is the treatment?

4. A 62 year old man suffers an anterior myocardial infarction but
makes an uneventful recovery. Eight days after the event he is
found extremely breathless and with a collapsed circulation.

Examination reveals a raised venous pressure and a new pansystolic
murmur heard throughout the praecordium. The ECG shows no
new changes and the chest X-ray shows bilateral diffuse opaci-
fication consistent with pulmonary oedema.

Questions:

1. What is the differential diagnosis?
2. What further investigations might you perform to make the
   diagnosis?

3. 1. Sub-aortic stenosis. The diagnosis is not hypertrophic obstructive cardiomyopathy because this would give a characteristic 'jerky' upstroke to the pulse.

2. Doppler echocardiography would show a gradient across the left ventricular outflow tract. Careful analysis of the cross-sectional echocardiogram will probably reveal the lesion especially if four chamber views are used.

3. The treatment depends on the degree of the obstruction and the type of sub-aortic stenosis diagnosed. There are broadly three types; membranous, fibromuscular and tunnel. The membranous type responds well to surgical excision, the fibromuscular form less so and the tunnel stenosis requires myomectomy and tends to recur.

4. 1. Post-infarction ventricular septal defect (VSD) or rupture of chordae or papillary muscle giving rise to severe mitral regurgitation.

2. Echocardiography preferably with colour flow doppler. Two dimensional echo may reveal the VSD but it is not reliable; colour flow doppler increases the sensitivity considerably. Echocardiography may show a flail mitral valve leaflet and doppler would reveal the degree of mitral regurgitation. However one must always exclude a VSD in these circumstances even if severe mitral regurgitation has been demonstrated. Therefore a right heart catheterisation recording the saturations is the investigation that must be performed if there is any doubt after echo/doppler studies. A saturation step-up in the pulmonary artery will be diagnostic.

5. A 56 year old woman presents to the medical out-patient depart-
    ment with a six-month history of increasing breathlessness on
    exertion, fatigue and an increase in weight. Her son who attends
    with her says that her voice has changed. She has never smoked. She
    had tuberculosis when she was 25 years old, successfully treated
    with streptomycin. Two years ago she had a debilitating flu-like
    illness with painful respiration and a tender chest wall.

    On examination she is obese with coarse features and a hoarse
    voice. Her pulse is 52/min regular with palpable paradox. The
    venous pressure is raised 10 cm with a prominent systolic descent.
    Heart sounds are soft but normal. The chest X-ray shows cardio-
    megaly with no other abnormalities.

    Questions:

    1. What is the diagnosis?
    2. What three possible underlying causes are there?
    3. What would your management be?
    4. What is the most likely cause of the illness two years ago?

6. A 52 year old Greek woman has a history of rheumatic fever. She is
    known to have mitral valve disease with mild shortness of breath on
    exertion which is said to be controlled with one tablet of Navidrex K
    daily. She takes no other regular medication. Three weeks ago she
    developed a chest infection productive of green sputum which was
    treated by the GP with amoxycillin. The infection appeared to clear
    but she became very breathless with orthopnoea, paroxysmal
    nocturnal dyspnoea and ankle swelling. Her sputum changed from
    green to white with flecks of blood.

    On examination the only positive physical findings were: a pulse of
    160/min irregularly irregular, blood pressure 100/70 mm Hg, venous
    pressure raised 4 cm, a loud first heart sound and a loud pulmonary
    component of the second heart sound and a long mid diastolic
    murmur. Fine and coarse inspiratory crackles could be heard in the
    chest and there was mild ankle oedema.

    Questions:

    1. What is the most likely cause for her deterioration?
    2. What underlying causes would you actively exclude?
    3. She was treated by the admitting houseman and within 24 hours
       was much improved. How had she treated her?

Answers overleaf

5. 1. Chronic pericardial effusion. The alternative diagnosis of constrictive pericarditis is unlikely because pulsus paradoxus is less common, the dominant venous pressure wave would be a rapid 'y' descent and the cardiac silhouette is rarely enlarged.

2. a. Myxoedema. This is the most likely cause in this case.

   b. Post-viral pericarditis. So-called idiopathic chronic pericardial effusions are probably the result of viral infection. Antibody titres in the pericardial fluid are often high. It commonly takes one to two years for a haemodynamically significant effusion to develop. It may cause a cholesterol pericarditis.

   c. Tuberculous pericarditis. This diagnosis should be considered but is the least likely of the three. Chronic tuberculous pericarditis commonly gives rise to pericardial calcification (which would show on X-ray) and constriction. It may produce a large chronic pericardial effusion but usually in less than 25 years.

3. Confirm the diagnosis on echocardiography. Tap the effusion. If it recurs refer for surgical drainage and pericardial window. Treat the underlying cause if appropriate.

4. Bornholm disease, resulting from Coxsackie B viral infection.

6. 1. Development of fast atrial fibrillation. The atrial component to ventricular filling becomes crucially important when there is restriction to ventricular inflow. Loss of the atrial component by fibrillation can make a critical difference. A chest infection is a common precipitating cause of atrial fibrillation.

2. Bacterial endocarditis and anaemia.

3. The heart rate was controlled with digoxin thus prolonging ventricular filling time.

7. You are asked to see a 60 year old man who has recovered from a prostatectomy eight days previously. He is known to have coronary artery disease and had quadruple coronary artery vein grafting three years ago. He normally takes diuretics. He has become suddenly short of breath and has a low blood pressure.

    On examination he is cold, clammy and pale. His pulse is regular at 100/min with a small volume and his blood pressure is 80/50 mm Hg. The venous pressure is 8 cm with a dominant 'a' wave and there is a fourth heart sound heard at the left sternal edge. Chest examination reveals no abnormalities.

    Questions:

    1. What is the diagnosis?
    2. What does the chest X-ray show?
    3. What would be the three mainstays of your initial management?

8. An 8 year old boy is referred to you with a heart murmur. He is otherwise well and there is nothing of note in the history.

    On examination he is a normal thin boy. Pulse is 90/min regular. Venous pressure is raised 1 cm with a dominant 'a' wave. There is a slight left parasternal heave and a systolic thrill felt at the left sternal edge. The first sound is normal and there is a soft second heart sound. There is an ejection click and a harsh ejection systolic murmur heard at the upper left sternal edge.

    The ECG shows sinus rhythm with right ventricular dominance and the chest X-ray shows pulmonary oligaemia.

    Questions:

    1. What is the diagnosis?
    2. Name one other feature which you would expect to see on chest x-ray.
    3. What is the treatment of choice?

Answers overleaf

7. 1. _Pulmonary embolus_. The timing of this episode is classical for pulmonary embolism which commonly occurs 7 to 14 days after an operation. There are frequently no clinical signs of deep vein thrombosis. The physical signs in this patient indicate right ventricular pressure overload which would not be in keeping with the alternative causes of post-operative collapse such as acute myocardial infarction, sepsis and blood loss.

2. An area of pulmonary oligaemia. It may also show collapse and possibly pulmonary oedema.

3. Oxygen therapy, intravenous plasma expanders (ideally plasma or blood) and anticoagulation.

8. 1. Pulmonary valvar stenosis. The clinical findings are typical of ventricular outflow tract obstruction, which is confirmed by the pulmonary oligaemia seen on right chest X-ray.

2. Post-stenotic dilatation of the pulmonary trunk.

3. Percutaneous balloon valvotomy. This non-surgical procedure is safe and effective in congenital non-calcified valvar pulmonary stenosis.

9. A 48 year old Indian presents to casualty with a two-hour history of pain in the back between the shoulder blades. It has not changed but has extended to involve the chest in the last 30 minutes. He smokes and has a family history of diabetes and ischaemic heart disease but has no previous illness other than hypertension treated for five years with atenolol.

On examination his pulse is 60/min, BP 110/50 mm Hg in the right arm and 160/50 mm Hg in the left arm. The venous pressure is raised 4 cm and the left carotid pulse is impalpable. The heart sounds are normal with a short immediate diastolic murmur at the left sternal edge.

The chest X-ray shows an enlarged cardiothoracic ratio and a wide mediastinum. The ECG shows sinus rhythm at 100/min. There is 3 mm ST segment elevation in leads II, III and aVF with T wave inversion in V5 and V6.

Questions:
1. What is the diagnosis?
2. Give two complications which have arisen.
3. How do you explain the physical findings?

10. A 65 year old man had an aortic valve replacement with a Bjork-Shiley prosthesis six months ago for mixed aortic valve disease. The post-operative course was complicated by the necessity to re-operate twice to stop bleeding, apparently from the aortic root cannula site. He is now admitted with a one-week history of breathlessness, fatigue and sweats. He is found to be pyrexial 38.5°C, with a venous pressure of 1 cm and a long early diastolic murmur. His white cell count is 18.9 x 10^9/l with a 97% neutrophilia, the ESR is 78 mm in the first hour. *Staphylococcus epidermidis* is grown from blood cultures and he is started on appropriate antibiotics.

He appears to be improving but three days later he deteriorates dramatically. On examination he is cold, sweaty and dusky blue. He is pyrexial 38°C. Pulse is 110/min, BP 100/40 mm Hg and the top of the venous pressure cannot be seen. The early diastolic murmur can be heard but there is a new continuous murmur heard at the left sternal edge.

Questions:
1. What was the diagnosis on admission?
2. Are you surprised at the organism that was isolated from the blood? Explain your reasons.
3. What happened to cause his dramatic deterioration?

Answers overleaf

9. 1. Acute dissection of the aorta.

2. Acute inferior myocardial infarction. Aortic regurgitation.

3. A dissection arising in the ascending aorta may follow a spiral course. In this patient compromised flow at the origin of the innominate artery results in a low blood pressure in the right arm; it has completely dissected the left common carotid origin but spared the left subclavian artery. The dissection of the aortic root has dilated the valve ring and caused aortic regurgitation. The raised venous pressure may result from the leakage into the pericardial sac or from right ventricular dysfunction following dissection of the right coronary artery and the consequent inferior infarction.

10. 1. Bacterial endocarditis involving the aortic valve prosthesis. One should be highly suspicious of an aortic root abscess given the complicated post-operative course.

2. No. *Staphylococcus epidermidis* is the most common organism causing early (within one year) prosthetic endocarditis.

3. The infection/abscess of the aortic root has caused the sinus of Valsalva to rupture into the right atrium. This accounts for the very high venous pressure which by distension of the systemic veins causes the apparent cyanosis. The communication between aorta and right atrium gives rise to the continuous murmur. This is a grave complication requiring immediate surgical correction.

CARDIOLOGY : DATA INTERPRETATIONS

1. This is the ECG of a man during exercise on a treadmill. He has reached stage II of a standard Bruce protocol.

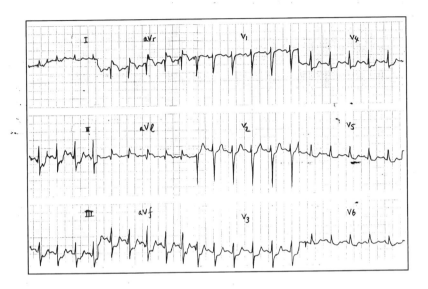

Questions:

1. What does the trace show?

2. How do you interpret the changes?

3. How would your management continue?

Answers overleaf

Data Interpretations : Answers

1. 1. There is ST segment depression greater than 1 mm 800 msec after the 'J' point in leads II, III. aVF and V3, V4, V5 and V6.

   2. Strongly positive exercise test. It suggests multi-vessel coronary disease because of the involvement of anterior and inferior leads.

   3. Define the coronary anatomy by cardiac catheterisation.

2. This is a 24 hour ST segment analysis in a man complaining of intermittent chest pain at rest.

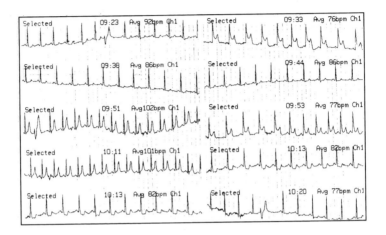

Questions:

1. What two features does it show?

2. What is the diagnosis?

2. 1. Intermittent ST segment elevation at 09.33 and 09.53, and ST depression at 10.13.

   2. Prinzmetal's angina or 'variant angina'. The ST segment elevation indicates acute sub-epicardial injury in contradistinction to ST segment depression which indicates sub-endocardial injury. Together they suggest significant coronary artery disease. Variant angina carries a poor prognosis and should always be investigated further.

3. These are pressure and saturation data resulting from cardiac catheterisation of a 22 year old woman.

Site	Pressure mm Hg	Saturation %
SVC	–	68
RA	6	78
RV	25/0–6	79
PA	25/8	80
LA	6	97
LV	110/0–5	96
AO	110/70	95

Questions:

1. What is the diagnosis?

2. What would your advice be?

4. These are pressure and saturation data resulting from cardiac catheterisation of a 52 year old woman with history of rheumatic fever who complains of severe breathlessness at rest and on exertion.

Site	Pressure mm Hg	Saturation %
RA	mean 13	65
RV	88/0–12	64
PA	85/40 mean 50	66
LA	mean 15	92
LV	120/0–6	91
Aorta	120/90	90

The cardiac output is measured at 3.4 litres per minute.

Questions:

1. What is the diagnosis?

2. What complication has arisen?

3. Is this lady a suitable surgical candidate?

Answers overleaf

3. 1. <u>Left to right shunt at atrial level</u>. This is most likely caused by an <u>artrial septal defect</u> but <u>anomalous pulmonary venous drainage is always possible.</u>

2. <u>Surgery would be the appropriate advice for a young woman with normal pulmonary artery pressure.</u> An ASD can allow <u>paradoxical emboli</u>, may become infected and if untreated the left to right shunt may lead to <u>pulmonary vascular disease</u> and <u>pulmonary hypertension</u> while the enlarging atria can lead to <u>supraventricular arrhythmias.</u> Closure of a secundum ASD is a relatively simple low risk procedure.

4. 1. <u>Mitral stenosis.</u> There is a <u>gradient between the left atrium and the end diastolic pressure in the left ventricle.</u>

2. <u>Pulmonary vascular disease and pulmonary hypertension.</u> There is a <u>significant pressure gradient across the pulmonary vascular bed (35 mm Hg)</u> which provides a considerable restriction to <u>flow in addition to the mitral valve disease. The pulmonary vascular resistance (PVR) in this patient has been calculated as 10 Wood units. PVR is the mean pressure difference between the pulmonary artery and the left atrium, divided by the cardiac output.</u>

3. The normal PVR is less than 1 and values greater than 8 carry a higher risk at surgery.

5. A 25 year old man has a systolic murmur noted at an insurance medical. The following are his catheter pressure data.

Site	Pressure mm Hg
RA	mean 0
RV	24/0–3
PA	24/12 mean 15
LA	mean 7
LV	220/0–8
Aorta	170/90
Femoral artery	90/60

Questions:

1. What is the diagnosis?

2. What associated lesion is present?

6. A 32 year old Jamaican woman complains of atypical chest pain. Investigation reveals a normal maximal exercise test but a routine blood test shows a serum triglyceride level of 2.7 mmol/l and a serum cholesterol level of 10.6 mmol/l.

Questions:

1. What is the diagnosis?

2. What treatment would you advise?

Answers overleaf

5. 1. Coarctation of the aorta.

2. Bicuspid aortic valve stenosis.

6. 1. Familial hypercholesterolaemia.

2. Low saturated fat diet with a bile acid sequestrant such as cholestyramine or a hydroxy-methyl-glutaryl coenzyme A reductase (HMG Co A) inhibitor such as simvastatin.

7. A 42 year old engineer has normal coronary arteries, no valvar regurgitation and the following angiographic measurements of left ventricular function.

End systolic volume 150 ml
End diastolic volume 180 ml
Ejection fraction 17%

Questions:

1. What is the diagnosis?

2. What are the therapeutic options?

8. After an acute inferior myocardial infarction in a 67 year old female the following intra-cardiac pressures were recorded with a Swan-Ganz catheter.

Site	Pressure mm Hg
RA	mean 8
RV	20/4–12
PA	18/5 mean 10
PA wedge	mean 4
Femoral artery	100/60

Question:

1. What is the explanation for these results?

Answers overleaf

7.   1. Dilated cardiomyopathy.

   2. Medical treatment would be directed at afterload reduction with angiotensin converting enzyme inhibitors pending cardiac transplantation.

8.   1. Right ventricular infarction with minimal damage to the left ventricle. The right ventricular filling pressure is very high while the left ventricular filling pressure is normal.

9. A man with hypertensive ischaemic heart disease was treated for an arrhythmia. He returned after syncopal episodes and this ECG was recorded.

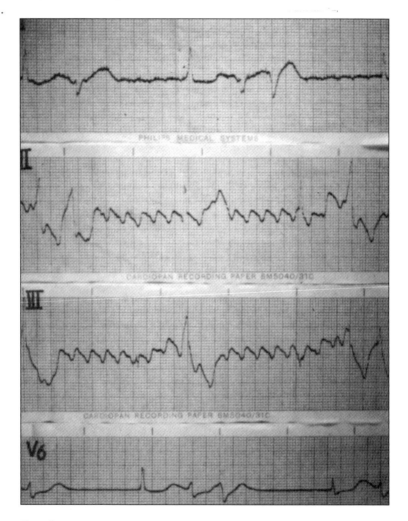

Questions:

1. What does the ECG show?

2. With what was the patient treated?

Answers overleaf

9. 1. Atrial flutter with a ventricular response rate of 30 per minute. This is complete heart block.

2. Digoxin.

Cardiology : Data Interpretations

10. This is the ECG of a 47 year old man with chest pain.

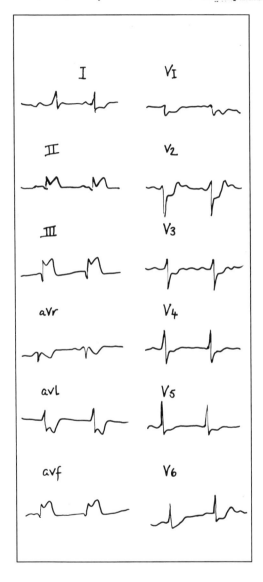

Question:

1. What does it show?

Answers overleaf
23

10.   1. Acute inferior myocardial infarction with posterior extension.

11. This ECG shows a self-terminating arrhythmia.

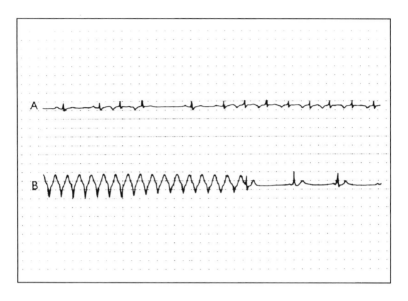

Question:

1. What is the underlying cause?

Answers overleaf

11. 1. Wolff-Parkinson-White syndrome.

12. A 65 year old male who lived alone was admitted to hospital having been found unconscious by his daughter. His medications, brought by his daughter, were atenolol, glyceryl trinitrate and sodium valproate.

Investigations included:

Serum creatine kinase	12,430 iu/l
aspartate aminotransferase	200 iu/l
hydroxybutyrate dehydrogenase	182 iu/l

ECG: normal

Questions:

1. What is the explanation for the findings?

2. What further investigation would you perform?

Answers overleaf

12. 1. There is a very large increase in creatine kinase levels which is unusually high for myocardial infarction in the absence of thrombolytic therapy. However, such levels are commonly found following a grand mal seizure, the most likely cause of this patient's collapse.

2. The creatine kinase iso-enzymes should be measured. If the MB fraction is low this will exclude myocardial infarction.

13. Study these three ECG traces. B was recorded 10 minutes after A and C four hours after B. (Trace C is illustrated overleaf.)

A

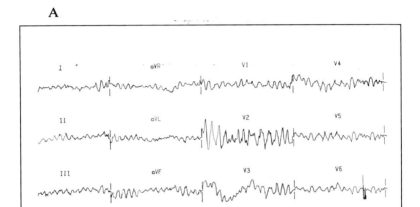

B

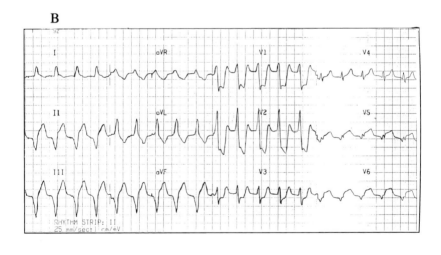

Continued overleaf

C

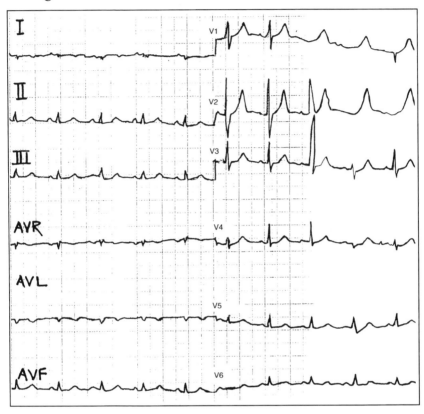

Questions:

1. What rhythm is shown in A?
2. What is the diagnosis in B?
3. What are the abnormalities seen in C?
4. What was done between B and C?

13. 1. Coarse ventricular fibrillation.

2. Hyperacute posterior myocardial infarction.

3. 'Q' waves and inverted 'T' waves in I and aVL; dominant 'R' wave and strongly positive 'T' wave in V1. Consistent with resolved posterior infarction.

4. The patient was treated with a thrombolytic agent, in this case intravenous streptokinase.

14. This is the ECG of a 60 year old man.

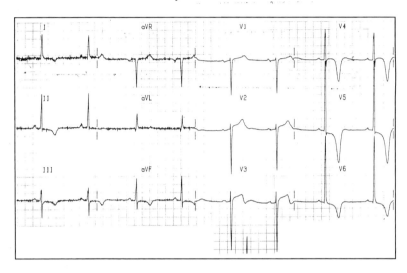

Questions:

1. How would you report this ECG?

2. What specific condition must be excluded?

Answers overleaf

14. 1. The ECG shows sinus rhythm at a rate of 50/min, the PR interval is 0.2 sec., the mean frontal QRS axis is within the normal range. The S wave in V2 added to the R wave in V5 is 72 mm. There is T wave inversion in leads I, II, III, aVL, aVF and chest leads V3-V6 with ST segment depression in V5 and V6. These features are consistent with left ventricular hypertrophy and strain. The lateral T wave inversion is so deep it is also consistent with recent lateral non-Q wave infarction.

2. Left ventricular outflow tract obstruction must be excluded by physical examination and echo/doppler studies.

15. This is an M-mode echocardiogram recorded at the level of the left ventricular cavity. The markers are one centimetre apart. Paper speed is 50 mm per second.

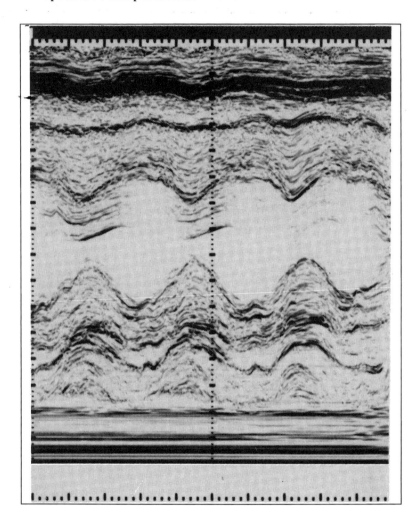

Question:

1. What does it show?

Answers overleaf

15. 1. The left ventricular cavity is small, the end systolic dimension is 2 cm (normal range 2.5–3.5) and the end diastolic dimension is 4.5 cm (normal range 3.5–5.0). The interventricular septum is 1.8 cm thick and the posterior wall 2.0 cm (upper limit of normal is 1.2 cm).

These findings reflect concentric left ventricular hypertrophy consistent with secondary ventricular hypertrophy and occasionally seen in non-obstructive hypertrophic cardiomyopathy.

16. This is the M-mode echocardiogram of a 25 year old woman recorded at the level of the aortic valve.

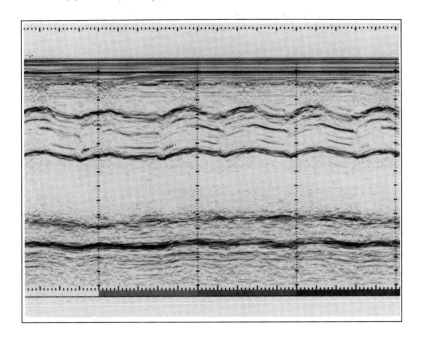

Question:

1. Comment on the left atrium and aortic valve leaflets?

16. 1. The left atrium is of normal size, the upper limit of normal being 4.0 cm. The aortic valve opens normally and there is low frequency flutter of the leaflets. This feature is normal. It should not be confused with high frequency flutter caused by turbulent flow which may be seen on normal aortic valve leaflets as a result of sub-aortic obstruction.

17. This is the M-mode echocardiogram of a 50 year old Italian woman, recorded at the level of the mitral valve.

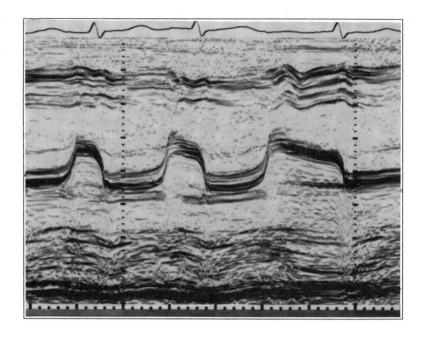

Questions:

1. What is the diagnosis?

2. What diagnostic features does it show?

17. 1. Mitral stenosis.

2. The characteristic features are thickening of the valve leaflets, anterior motion of the posterior valve leaflet, delayed closure of the valve without the normal mid diastolic closure. This is reflected in the filling of the ventricle which fills throughout diastole. This can be clearly seen from the septal echoes.

18. This is the electrocardiogram of a 40 year old man who gives one-week history of feeling non-specifically unwell. One hour prior to admission he vomited and collapsed. His wife managed to bring him to casualty where this trace was taken.

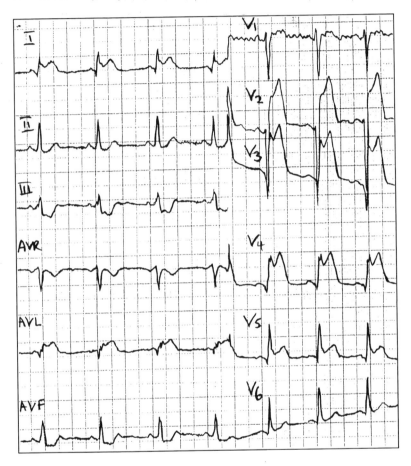

Questions:

1. What does the ECG show?

2. What is the anatomical basis for what is seen?

3. What would be the treatment of choice?

Answers overleaf

18. 1. Sinus rhythm with ST segment elevation in anterior and lateral leads and segment depression in inferior leads. This is consistent with the hyperacute changes of an anterior infarction.

      2. Anterior infarction is caused by occlusion of the left anterior descending artery.

      3. The history with the ECG findings suggests very recent occlusion of the artery and immediate thrombolytic therapy would be most appropriate.

19. This is the electrocardiogram of a 35 year old woman with a history of palpitations.

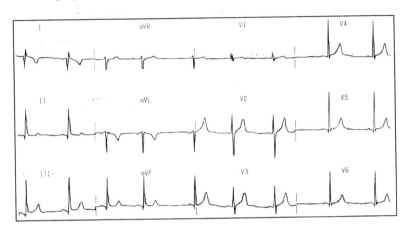

Question:

1. What is the cause of the abnormality shown in this ECG?

19. 1. The abnormality noted is the 'P' wave axis which appears greater than 110°. This is not an abnormal atrial focus however. The limb leads aVR and aVL have been accidentally interchanged. The revised trace would be normal.

20. The following pressure recordings were taken from cardiac catheterisation data on a 14 year old cyanosed boy.

Site   Pressure mm Hg

RA   mean 8
RV   120/0–8
PA   mean 20
LV   110/0–8
Aorta   110/60 mean 85

Question:

1. What two anatomical defects could account for this data?

20. 1. The data suggests supra-systemic right ventricular pressures but almost normal pulmonary artery pressures. This can only be the case if there is severe right ventricular outflow tract obstruction, for example due to pulmonary stenosis or infundibular stenosis. However, pulmonary stenosis would not alone account for the cyanosis so there must be right to left shunting occurring at ventricular level. The two anatomical defects are therefore right ventricular outflow tract obstruction and ventricular septal defect.

RESPIRATORY MEDICINE : CASE HISTORIES

1. A 48 year old man smoked 20 cigarettes daily and had been breathless on exertion for a number of years. He presented with increased breathlessness and cough productive of yellow sputum following a cold one week previously. His general practitioner had prescribed a salbutamol aerosol but this had produced no subjective improvement. His father had a 'bad chest' and his brother aged 45 had recently been admitted to hospital with a similar problem.

On examination he was breathless at rest and cyanosed. There was no finger clubbing nor signs of heart failure but his chest was hyperexpanded, with quiet wheezes and a few early inspiratory basal crackles.

Investigations showed:

Arterial blood (breathing air):
PO_2	6.8 kPa (51 mm Hg)
PCO_2	5.9 kPa (44 mm Hg)
pH	7.36
Bicarbonate	24 mmol/l
Hb	12.5 g/dl
WBC	14.6 x 10^9/l, 80% granulocytes, 10% lymphocytes, 6% monocytes

Peak expiratory flow rate: unrecordable.

Chest radiograph: increased lung volumes and increased radiolucency in both lower zones.

Questions:

1. Give four diagnoses which could account for his dyspnoea.

2. Give four measures which should be undertaken in his immediate treatment.

Answers overleaf

1. 1. Chronic airflow limitation (CAL) (chronic obstructive lung disease, chronic obstructive airways disease) resulting from cigarette smoking is likely to be important. His relatively young age, family history of chest disease, and increased radiolucency in both lower zones (which might represent bulla formation) are features which raise the possibility of emphysema due to alpha-1-antitrypsin deficiency.

In spite of the lack of subjective response to salbutamol, his symptoms and the family history also raises the possibility of asthma either as the sole diagnosis or in addition to CAL.

The coloured sputum and polymorphonuclear leucocytosis further suggest a lower respiratory tract infection as the cause of the recent exacerbation of his breathlessness.

A bronchial carcinoma in the proximal airways, not apparent on chest radiograph, is another possible diagnosis particularly when there is a poor response to therapy.

2. Oxygen will be required in view of his hypoxaemia. The aim should be to elevate the PaO_2 to at least 7.5 kPa (55 mm Hg) since values less than this fall on the steep part of the oxygen-haemoglobin dissociation curve and are therefore associated with substantial haemoglobin desaturation. Bronchodilator therapy, corticosteroids, and antibiotics should be given.

2. A 62 year old man who smoked 30 cigarettes daily had intermittent episodes of minor haemoptysis for several years, but during the previous two weeks had produced a cupful of blood on four occasions. He also gave a history of longstanding breathlessness on exertion and daily productive cough. He had pulmonary tuberculosis as a young man.

No abnormality was found on examination but his chest radiograph showed right apical streaky shadowing.

Investigations showed:

Hb	11.9 g/dl
WBC	$8.4 \times 10^9/l$
ESR	30 mm in the first hour
Liver function tests: normal	
FEV_1	1.9 l (predicted 2.3–3.4)
FVC	3.0 l (predicted 3.1–4.6)
FEV_1/FVC	63%

Fibreoptic bronchoscopy demonstrated no abnormality and bronchial washings were negative for acid and alcohol fast bacilli and malignant cells.

Computed tomography (CT) scanning of the chest demonstrated right apical shadowing compatible with fibrosis, and a cavity within which there was a 2 cm mass. The mediastinum was normal.

Questions:

1. What are the two most likely causes of this man's haemoptysis?

2. How would you manage this case?

Answers overleaf

2. 1. Aspergilloma and bronchial carcinoma are the two most likely diagnoses, the former being more probable in this case.

2. Serum precipitins to *Aspergillus fumigatus* should be measured since these are usually strongly positive in patients with an aspergilloma. The fungus ball is commonly mobile within the cavity, as can be demonstrated by CT scanning with the patient prone and supine. If malignancy remains a possibility percutaneous needle biopsy is indicated.

   The patient has had four major haemoptyses and is at risk for a life-threatening haemorrhage. Surgical resection of an aspergilloma which is causing such severe bleeding is the treatment of choice. In cases where this is not feasible, selective bronchial artery embolisation, radiotherapy, and inhaled or intracavitary antifungal agents have all been tried with varying degrees of success. If the lesion is a carcinoma, it should be staged and treated appropriately.

3. A 63 year old man who smoked ten cigarettes daily presented with a four-year history of breathlessness. During the previous two months his breathlessness had been worse and associated with left sided chest pain. He had never taken any regular medication nor had he kept any pets. He had worked as a stoker in the merchant navy for ten years as a young man.

On examination he had finger clubbing and wheezes. At the right lung base there were late inspiratory crackles, and at the left base there was dullness to percussion and reduced breath sounds. His chest radiograph showed right basal shadowing and diaphragmatic calcification, and there was a moderate left pleural effusion.

Investigations showed:

Hb	13.5 g/dl
WBC	$7.6 \times 10^9/l$
ESR	30 mm in the first hour
FEV_1	1.9 l (predicted 2.5–3.8)
FVC	3.1 l (predicted 3.4–5.1)
FEV_1/FVC	61%

Total lung capacity: 5.0 l (predicted 5.4–8.1)
Transfer coefficient for carbon monoxide: 0.9 mmol/min/kPa/l (predicted 1.2–1.7)

Questions:

1. What two main abnormalities are revealed by the lung function tests?

2. What is the most likely underlying cause of the clinical abnormalities?

3.　1.　The combination of a reduction in FEV_1 and FVC and reduction in FEV_1/FVC% indicates the presence of airflow limitation.

The reduction in TLC indicates the presence of a restrictive defect. Since the KCO is low, the restrictive defect is likely to be due, at least in part, to parenchymal lung disease although the pleural effusion would also contribute.

2.　Asbestos related lung disease; previous asbestos exposure is suggested by the diaphragmatic calcification, and history of work as a stoker (during which there was often close contact with asbestos lagged pipes and boilers). Asbestos exposure may cause asbestosis which could explain this patient's restrictive defect, crackles, and clubbing. Mesothelioma and bronchial carcinoma are likely causes of his pleural effusion since asbestos exposure predisposes to both of these. Cigarette smoking would account for his airflow limitation.

4. A 33 year old woman had pneumonia as a child. She subsequently had several episodes each year of cough productive of yellow sputum which were treated with courses of antibiotics. These episodes became more frequent and by the age of 30 she had a daily cough productive of yellow sputum and developed breathlessness with wheeze on substantial exertion such as climbing more than 20 stairs. She also had persistent rhinorrhoea and recurrent sinusitis. She had never smoked cigarettes. Her mother had a similar complaint. On examination there were wheezes and bilateral early inspiratory crackles.

Investigations showed:

Chest radiograph: bilateral basal shadowing with thickened bronchial walls and ring shadows.

Hb	12.6 g/dl
WBC	5.7 x 10^9/l
ESR	30 mm in the first hour

Fibreoptic bronchoscopy showed purulent secretions in the basal segments of both lower lobes.

Questions:

1. What diagnosis would account for her productive cough?

2. What three investigations would you undertake to demonstrate the underlying cause?

3. What is the likely cause of her wheeze?

Answers overleaf

4. 1. Bronchiectasis. This diagnosis is suggested by the history of chronic cough productive of coloured sputum, and the chest radiograph appearances.

2. In many patients no underlying cause will be apparent. However, measurement of serum immunoglobulins is important to exclude hypogammaglobulinaemia which can present with recurrent respiratory infections and subsequent bronchiectasis. A skin sweat test will help exclude cystic fibrosis which can present in this age group. Assessment of ciliary function, which may require referral to a specialist centre, will be necessary to exclude primary ciliary dyskinesia (which includes Kartagener's syndrome). Other important causes of bronchiectasis include severe pneumonia, and bronchial obstruction (with subsequent distal infection) of which there was no evidence at bronchoscopy in this patient.

3. Her wheeze is probably due to asthma which is more common in patients with bronchiectasis, and which should be treated in the usual way.

5. A 27 year old woman gave a three day history of painful swallowing and sore throat. The day prior to presentation she noted that she was breathless on carrying the shopping and her breathing was noisy. Her general practitioner had prescribed amoxycillin capsules but she was otherwise taking no regular medication. She had asthma as a child and there was a family history of asthma.

    On examination she was febrile (38°C) and there was stridor. There was no abnormality of the mouth or fauces, her chest was clear, and the remainder of the examination was normal.

    Investigations showed:

    Hb   12.6 g/dl
    WBC   15.6 x 10⁹/l, 70% granulocytes, 21% lymphocytes, 9% monocytes

    Peak expiratory flow rate 280 l/min (predicted 420–680)

    Chest radiograph: normal

    Questions:

    1. What is the most likely diagnosis?

    2. List four important steps in the management of this patient.

Answers overleaf

5. 1. Acute epiglottitis is suggested by the recent onset of painful swallowing, sore throat, and stridor. Although uncommon in adults, it is important to recognise this condition quickly since fatal airway obstruction may occur with little warning.

2. Urgent confirmation of the diagnosis is required by laryngoscopy by an ENT surgeon. This procedure can be performed with relative safety in adults in whom it is unlikely to provoke laryngospasm. Although lateral soft tissue X-rays of the neck may demonstrate swelling of the epiglottis, this is a time consuming investigation in these circumstances and definitive diagnosis will require laryngoscopy in any case.

The airway should be safeguarded urgently either by tracheostomy or endotracheal intubation, and humidification should be provided. Corticosteroids may subsequently be used with the aim of controlling local oedema. Intravenous antibiotics should be given since the most common recognised cause of epiglottitis is haemophilus influenzae type B. This organism is now frequently resistant to ampicillin so chloramphenicol or an appropriate cephalosporin, such as cefuroxime, is preferable.

6. A 26 year old man had been injecting heroin intravenously for two years. He presented with a three-month history of night sweats, malaise, increasing breathlessness and recently, a cough productive of small amounts of clear sputum. There was no history of cardiac disease, he took no regular medication other than heroin, and had not travelled abroad for over five years.

On examination he was febrile (38.5°C). There were injection marks in his arms. He had oral candidiasis and enlarged slightly tender cervical, axillary, and inguinal lymph nodes. There were a few basal crackles but no other signs in the chest.

Investigations showed:

Hb   12.6 g/dl
WBC 4.2 x 10^9/l

Chest radiograph: normal

Arterial blood: (breathing air)

PO_2 9.0 kPa (68 mm Hg)
PCO_2 4.1 kPa (31 mm Hg)

Questions:

1. What is the most likely underlying cause for this man's clinical presentation?

2. What is the probable cause of his respiratory symptoms?

3. What measures should be undertaken in the management of the pulmonary pathology?

Answers overleaf

6. 1. Infection by the human immunodeficiency virus (HIV) is suggested by the presence of generalised lymphadenopathy and oral candidiasis in an intravenous drug abuser.

2. In industrialised countries, over half of patients with HIV infection who develop the acquired immunodeficiency syndrome (AIDS), present with pneumonia due to *Pneumocystis carinii* infection which is the most likely cause of the respiratory symptoms in this patient. The chest radiograph characteristically shows bilateral diffuse lung shadowing but other appearances, including patchy shadowing, may be seen. Alternatively the radiograph may be normal. Pulmonary involvement by cytomegalovirus, myco- and other bacteria must also be considered but are less common causes. Kaposi's sarcoma involving the lungs occurs in HIV infected patients but characteristically causes nodular rather than diffuse shadowing on the chest radiograph and is more likely to occur in homosexuals than intravenous drug abusers with AIDS.

3. Sputum should be examined by routine Gram stain, and specifically for *Pneumocystis carinii* and acid fast bacilli. Routine bacteriological culture, and culture for mycobacteria, should be requested. Nebulized hypertonic saline may be necessary to help obtain sputum in individuals in whom it is sparse. If samples are not available or results are negative, most centres perform early fibreoptic bronchoscopy with bronchoalveolar lavage and transbronchial biopsy. Some centres treat empirically and proceed to bronchoscopy only if the patient's condition is not improving.

If a diagnosis of *P. carinii* pneumonia is confirmed, treatment should be started with high dose cotrimoxazole.

7. A 46 year old man presented with a two-month history of dry cough. He had no other respiratory symptoms but had noted that he was having nose bleeds more frequently than before. Five months previously he had developed a skin rash on both feet which was investigated at another hospital where a skin biopsy had been done, but the patient had failed to attend for follow up. There was no personal nor family history of asthma and he was taking no regular medication.

On examination there was a faint macular skin rash on both feet but no abnormality in the respiratory system and the remainder of the examination was normal. Enquiries were made into the results of the skin biopsy and this was found to have demonstrated vasculitis with infiltration by mononuclear cells.

Investigations showed:

Hb   14.6 g/dl
WBC   5.7 x 10^9/l, 65% neutrophils,1% eosinophils,
            21% lymphocytes,10% monocytes
ESR   60 mm in the first hour

Plasma sodium	132 mmol/l
potassium	4.2 mmol/l
urea	11.0 mmol/l
creatinine	180 μmol/l

Chest radiograph: bilateral patchy shadowing predominantly in the mid zones, with some cavitation.

Questions:

1. What are the three most likely diagnoses?

2. What three investigations would you perform to establish the diagnosis?

Answers overleaf

7. 1. This patient could have a systemic vasculitis affecting skin, lungs and (in view of the elevated plasma urea and creatinine) kidneys. The principal causes of systemic vasculitis producing abnormality on the chest radiograph are Wegener's granulomatosis, polyarteritis nodosa (PAN) and the Churg-Strauss syndrome. The history of epistaxis, cavitation of lung shadows, renal impairment and mononuclear cell infiltrate suggests Wegener's granulomatosis. In PAN neutrophils are characteristically the predominant cell in the inflammatory infiltrate. In the Churg-Strauss syndrome the kidneys are usually spared and the predominant inflammatory cell is the eosinophil.

2. Examination by an ENT surgeon may reveal abnormalities of the upper respiratory tract in Wegener's granulomatosis, including ulcerating lesions of the nasal septum, palate, sinuses or pharynx. Although this patient has already had a skin biopsy, a further biopsy would provide histological confirmation of organ involvement by vasculitis; thus fibreoptic bronchoscopy with transbronchial biopsy, or renal biopsy, would be helpful. Mesenteric or renal angiography may demonstrate small aneurysms and vessels blocked by thrombi in PAN but this investigation has low sensitivity.

8. A 53 year old man who smoked 40 cigarettes daily and had a longstanding daily cough productive of white sputum, presented with a three-month history of intermittent haemoptysis. There was no significant medical history and he was taking no regular medication. In his twenties he had spent four years lagging pipes and subsequently worked in the building trade.

On examination he had finger clubbing and a hard 1 cm lymph node in the right supraclavicular fossa. There were no signs in the chest and no hepatomegaly.

Investigations showed:

Hb   13.6 g/dl
WBC   5.7 x 10⁹/l
Serum   bilirubin   28 μmol/l
        glutamic-oxaloacetic transaminase 65 iu/l
        alkaline phosphatase   194 iu/l (normal
                                                          40–100)

Chest radiograph: a 3 cm mass in the right mid zone and bilateral diaphragmatic calcification.

Questions:

1. What is the most likely diagnosis and what two factors might have contributed to its development?

2. List four investigations which may confirm the diagnosis.

3. Having made the diagnosis, how would you manage this patient?

Answers overleaf

8. 1. The finger clubbing and radiological findings suggest that this patient has a bronchial carcinoma. Clubbing is particularly associated with bronchial adenocarcinoma and squamous carcinoma. The likely aetiological factors include his cigarette smoking and asbestos exposure; these two have a multiplicative effect in increasing the chance of developing a bronchial carcinoma.

2. The enlarged lymph node and abnormal liver function probably represent metastatic spread from a bronchial carcinoma; needle aspiration of the lymph node for cytological examination, or excision biopsy, provides a rapid and simple method of diagnosis. Alternatively, the sputum may be examined for malignant cells. If the diagnosis were not obtained by these means it would be necessary to undertake fibreoptic bronchoscopy and biopsy. If this examination were normal, a percutaneous needle biopsy might reveal positive results.

3. A non-oat cell bronchial carcinoma, in this patient who has evidence of distant metastasis, would be treated by palliative radiotherapy for the haemoptysis. Oat cell bronchial carcinoma may be treated with chemotherapy.

9. A 35 year old woman from Nigeria who had never smoked cigarettes presented with intermittent cough and haemoptysis which had started about ten years previously. There was no dyspnoea, sputum production, nor chest pain. Her symptoms had been investigated in her home country with blood tests and chest radiographs but no diagnosis had been made and no results of these investigations were available. She had taken the oral contraceptive pill for a period of five years starting at the age of 22 but at the time of her presentation was taking no regular medication, and there was no history of deep venous thrombosis.

Examination was normal with no signs in the respiratory system.

Investigations showed:

Hb   12.5 g/dl
WBC   7.6 X 10^9/l
Platelets   240 x 10^9/l
ESR   15 mm in the first hour
Prothrombin time 14 seconds (control 14)

Chest radiograph: normal

Questions:

1. Give three possible causes of her haemoptysis.

2. What three investigations should be undertaken to make a diagnosis?

Answers overleaf

9. 1. A slow growing bronchial neoplasm such as a bronchial carcinoid may be responsible and can be associated with a normal chest radiograph. Such tumours may undergo malignant change. A localised area of bronchiectasis can cause recurrent haemoptysis without radiographic abnormality and is not always associated with the production of mucopurulent sputum. It is unusual for pulmonary emboli to present with recurrent haemoptysis alone, over such a long time span, but this diagnosis should be considered. Hereditary haemorrhagic telangiectasia (Osler-Rendu-Weber syndrome) is a rare cause of recurrent haemoptysis. As a general rule recurrent haemoptysis is an unlikely mode of presentation for a bleeding disorder and in any case this patient's platelet count and prothrombin time are normal.

   2. Fibreoptic bronchoscopy may reveal an endobronchial lesion such as a bronchial carcinoid tumour. Computerised tomography scanning may provide evidence of a localised abnormality such as bronchiectasis and, if necessary, this diagnosis could be confirmed by bronchography. A ventilation perfusion isotope lung scan would be helpful in excluding pulmonary emboli.

10. A 49 year old man, a lifelong non-smoker, presented with recurrent episodes of cough productive of purulent sputum for approximately ten years. There was no dyspnoea, chest pain, or haemoptysis, and he was well between episodes. There was no personal history of other illness and there was no family history of a similar complaint. A routine chest radiograph twenty years previously was apparently abnormal but he could not remember what diagnosis had been made.

On examination breath sounds were slightly reduced over the left lung but there was no abnormality of the chest wall and the remainder of the examination was normal.

Investigations showed:

Hb	13.8 g/dl
WBC	5.4 x 10^9/l
FEV_1	2.7 l (predicted 2.8–4.2)
FVC	4.1 l (predicted 3.7–5.5)
FEV_1/FVC	66%

Chest radiograph: hypertransradiancy of left lung with some mediastinal shift to the left.

Questions:

1. What is the most probable diagnosis? List three other possibilities which need to be excluded.

2. List two investigations which will support the diagnosis.

Answers overleaf

10. 1. Provided there is no chest wall abnormality and the chest radiograph is well centred, this radiographic appearance is suggestive of Macleod's syndrome in which there is unilateral hypertransradiancy due to hypoplasia of the affected lung with a small pulmonary artery and fewer alveoli. There is usually evidence of mild airflow limitation. The mediastinum may be central, or shifted towards the affected lung. Conditions which can cause a similar appearance include emphysema (bullous or compensatory), obstructive over-inflation (in which the mediastinum would be shifted away from the affected side), and pulmonary embolus (which is likely to be distinguished on clinical grounds).

2. An expiratory chest radiograph may show shift of the mediastinum away from the affected side due to air trapping. An isotope ventilation perfusion lung scan will show reduced perfusion and ventilation, in contrast to the mismatch of ventilation and perfusion which is seen in pulmonary embolism.

RESPIRATORY MEDICINE : DATA INTERPRETATIONS

1. An obese 56 year old woman complains of daytime somnolence. Her husband says that she snores loudly.

   Investigations showed:

   Arterial blood (breathing air):

PO_2	10.4 kPa (78 mm Hg)
PCO_2	5.6 kPa (42 mm Hg)

   Questions:

   1. What is the most likely diagnosis?

   2. How can this diagnosis be confirmed?

2. A 60 year old woman is prescribed indomethacin for osteoarthritis and six weeks later returns complaining of breathlessness.

   Investigations showed:

   Chest radiograph: normal
   FEV_1 2.9 l (predicted 2.5–3.2)
   FVC   3.9 l (predicted 3.4–4.2)
   FEV_1/FVC   74%

   Question:

   1. List three possible causes of her increased breathlessness.

Answers overleaf

1. 1. <u>Sleep apnoea</u>, which is commoner in <u>obese</u> patients. There is <u>nocturnal hypoxaemia</u> but daytime arterial blood gases may be normal.

    2. The presence of sleep apnoeas and whether these are central or obstructive can be determined by <u>overnight polysomnography</u>. This may include oximetry, measurement of nasal and oral airflow, electroencephalography, and electromyography.

2. 1. <u>Sensitivity to indomethacin or other non-steroidal anti-inflammatory drugs may cause the appearance of, or deterioration in, asthma in susceptible subjects. The normal lung function tests do not exclude this diagnosis since bronchospasm may be intermittent.</u>

    <u>Fluid retention</u> and pulmonary congestion may be caused by non-steroidal anti-inflammatory drugs.

    <u>Anaemia secondary to gastrointestinal bleeding</u> induced by indomethacin.

3. A 53 year old previously healthy man presents with a two-week history of lethargy and cough productive of yellow sputum. Chest radiograph demonstrates patchy consolidation in both lower zones.

    Investigations showed:

Hb	8.7 g/dl
Reticulocyte count	4.2%
WBC	9.3 x 10⁹/l

    Questions:

    1. What is the probable diagnosis?

    2. What three tests would confirm this diagnosis, and what treatment would you give for it?

4. A 74 year old man presents with a two-month history of lethargy and breathlessness. He has hepatosplenomegaly, generalised lymphadenopathy, and a left pleural effusion, aspiration of which reveals straw coloured fluid.

    Investigations showed:

    Pleural fluid:
    Protein: 46 g/l
    Cytology: abundant lymphocytes
    Gram stain: no bacteria
    Routine culture: no bacterial growth
    Stain for alcohol acid fast bacilli: negative

Hb	12.6 g/dl
WBC	56.4 x 10⁹/l, 92% lymphocytes, 6% granulocytes, 2% monocytes
ESR	120 mm in the first hour

    Questions:

    1. List two likely causes of the pleural effusion.

    2. Give three investigations which may be helpful in determining the cause of the effusion.

Answers overleaf

Data Interpretations : Answers

3. 1. The clinical picture is suggestive of infection with *Mycoplasma pneumoniae* which can produce both pneumonia and haemolytic anaemia (the latter due to cold agglutinins).

2. The diagnosis of *Mycoplasma pneumoniae* would be supported by the demonstration of a positive direct Coomb's antiglobulin test, cold agglutinins in the serum, and complement fixing antibodies to *M. pneumoniae* in paired sera. The infection responds to treatment with erythromycin or tetracycline.

4. 1. The haematological indices suggest chronic lymphocytic leukaemia. Likely causes of the lymphocytic pleural effusion therefore include leukaemic infiltration or pulmonary tuberculosis. Tuberculous pleural effusions yield fluid which is often negative on Ziehl Nielsen stain, but which characteristically contain increased numbers of lymphocytes.

2. A pleural biopsy should be obtained for histology. This, and pleural fluid, should also be cultured for mycobacteria. Lymphocytes in a pleural effusion caused by leukaemic infiltration may have a characteristic morphological appearance, and/or surface markers as determined by immunophenotyping.

70

5. A 48 year old man with advanced Hodgkin's lymphoma (stage IIIB) is receiving cytotoxic chemotherapy with cyclophosphamide, vinblastine, procarbazine, and prednisolone. He becomes breathless and his chest radiograph shows bilateral lung shadowing predominantly in the mid zones.

Investigations showed:

Hb   8.5 g/dl
WBC $1.5 \times 10^9/l$, 70% granulocytes, 16% lymphocytes, 14% monocytes
Platelets $95 \times 10^9/l$

Questions:

1. List three likely causes of the lung shadowing.

2. What further investigation might help distinguish between these causes?

6. A 66 year old man who smokes 20 cigarettes daily presents with a two-week history of lethargy and haemoptysis. Chest radiograph shows shadowing in the right mid and lower zones.

Investigations showed:

Plasma sodium	134 mmol/l
potassium	5.2 mmol/l
bicarbonate	18 mmol/l
urea	35 mmol/l
Serum creatinine	410 μmol/l

Question:

1. List three diagnoses, each of which could account for these findings.

Answers overleaf

5. 1. The patient is likely to be immunodeficient as a result of both the lymphoma itself, and the immunosuppressive drug therapy. *Pneumocystis carinii*, cytomegalovirus, Mycobacterium tuberculosis and other bacteria and fungi may cause pulmonary infections in immunocompromised subjects. A number of cytotoxic drugs, including cyclophosphamide, may cause pneumonitis and pulmonary fibrosis. The pulmonary shadowing may also be caused by infiltration of the lungs by lymphoma, which occurs in 30–40% of patients with Hodgkin's disease, particularly the nodular sclerosing type.

2. Fibreoptic bronchoscopy, with bronchoalveolar lavage and transbronchial biopsy, or open lung biopsy. These should be done early in the illness.

6. 1. There are a number of possible causes of haemoptysis and renal impairment. Bronchial carcinoma, and other tumours, may be associated with membranous glomerulonephritis. In Goodpasture's syndrome there are antibodies to glomerular and alveolar basement membrane. Renal impairment may occur in pneumonia caused by *Legionella pneumophila* or *Mycoplasma pneumoniae*. Systemic vasculitides may affect both lung and kidneys, particularly polyarteritis nodosa and Wegener's granulomatosis.

7. A 35 year old woman who has never smoked cigarettes is investigated for vitiligo and the recent onset of lethargy and breathlessness. She is found to have autoimmune hypoadrenalism.

Investigations showed:

FEV$_1$ 1.9 (predicted 2.5–3.4)
FVC   3.5 (predicted 3.5–4.3)
FEV$_1$/FVC 54%

Questions:

1. What is the likely cause of her breathlessness?

2. How would you confirm this diagnosis?

8. An 81 year old man who smokes 30 cigarettes daily presents with a three-month history of haemoptysis. He has finger clubbing and the chest radiograph demonstrates a cavitating shadow in the left lower lobe.

Investigations showed:

Serum calcium   3.4 mmol/l
         phosphate   1.2 mmol/l

Questions:

1. What is the probable diagnosis?

2. What treatment is most appropriate for the haemoptysis?

Answers overleaf

7. 1. The reduced FEV_1 and FEV_1/FVC ratio indicate the presence of airflow limitation which in a young non-smoker is likely to be due to asthma. In a susceptible subject the onset of hypoadrenalism may precipitate the development of asthma, which is likely to respond to adequate corticosteroid replacement therapy.

2. The diagnosis of asthma depends on demonstrating variability in airflow limitation. This may occur spontaneously (conveniently demonstrated by serial recordings of peak expiratory flow rate), with a bronchodilator, or (in patients in whom FEV_1 is at least 60% of predicted volume) following bronchoconstrictors such as methacholine or histamine in a bronchial provocation test.

8. 1. Bronchial carcinoma. The combination of finger clubbing, cavitation on chest radiograph, and hypercalcaemia is more commonly seen with squamous cell tumours than with other types of bronchial carcinoma.

2. Radiotherapy.

9. A 36 year old woman gave birth to her first child and two weeks later presented with breathlessness at rest. Examination and chest radiograph were normal.

Investigations showed:

Hb   13.4 g/dl
FEV_1 2.6 l (predicted 2.4–3.6)
FVC   3.6 l (predicted 3.1–4.6)
FEV_1/FVC   72%
Arterial blood (breathing air):
   PO_2 8.3 kPa (62 mm Hg)
   PCO_2 3.5 kPa (26 mm Hg)
   pH   7.44

Questions:

1. What is the most likely diagnosis?

2. How would you confirm this diagnosis?

10. A 20 year old woman with hayfever presents with a six-month history of daily unproductive cough which is worse at night and going out into cold air. She does not wheeze and has never smoked cigarettes. Examination and chest radiograph are normal.

Investigations showed:

Peak expiratory flow rate 410 l/min (predicted 340–500)
FEV_1 2.9 l (predicted 2.4–3.6)
FVC   3.8 l (predicted 2.6–4.0)
FEV_1/FVC 76%

Questions:

1. What is the most likely diagnosis?

2. How would you confirm this diagnosis?

3. What would be your management?

Answers overleaf

9. 1. Pulmonary thromboembolism. This is associated with preg-
   nancy, can cause breathlessness in the absence of abnormality on
   physical examination or chest radiograph, and would account for
   the hypoxaemia (caused by ventilation-perfusion mismatch).

   2. In pulmonary embolism, ventilation (V) and perfusion (Q)
   isotope lung scanning will demonstrate perfusion defects which
   are not matched by ventilation defects (i.e. V/Q mismatch).

10. 1. Asthma. Cough may be the only symptom and, in common with
   other symptoms of asthma, is particularly liable to occur at night.
   The absence of findings on physical examination and normal
   lung function is compatible with this diagnosis.

   2. Increased variability in airflow limitation may be demonstrated
   by serial recordings of peak expiratory flow rate, or by testing
   before and after a bronchodilator. Bronchial provocation (for
   example with histamine or methacholine) may be used to
   demonstrate airway hyperresponsiveness, which is the hallmark
   of asthma.

   3. If the diagnosis of asthma is confirmed, anti-asthma treatment
   should be given. If the cough does not respond to this, and there
   is no evidence of nasal sinus or laryngeal disease, fibreoptic
   bronchoscopy will be required to exclude an endobronchial
   lesion (such as an inhaled foreign body or bronchial neoplasm)
   which is a less likely underlying cause in this patient.

11. A 68 year old man presented with longstanding progressively worsening breathlessness on exertion. He smoked 30 cigarettes daily and on examination was wheezy.

Investigations showed:

FEV$_1$ 1.5 l (predicted 2.1–3.1)
FVC   2.9 l (predicted 3.0–4.4)
FEV$_1$/FVC   52%
Total lung capacity (TLC) 7.0 l (predicted 4.9–7.4)
Transfer factor for carbon monoxide (TLCO) 5.5 mmol/min/kPa
  (predicted 6.4–9.6)
Transfer coefficient for carbon monoxide (KCO)
  0.85 mmol/min/kPa/l (predicted 1.1–1.6)
Hb 17.8 g/dl

Question:

1. What is the diagnosis?

12. A 53 year old man who has never smoked cigarettes presents with a six-month history of breathlessness. On examination there is finger clubbing and at the base of each lung crackles. Chest radiograph demonstrates bilateral basal shadowing.

Investigations showed:

FEV$_1$ 2.2 l (predicted 2.5–3.7)
FVC   2.7 l (predicted 3.3–4.9)
FEV$_1$/FVC   81%
Total lung capacity (TLC) 4.8 l (predicted 5.0–7.5)
Transfer factor for carbon monoxide (TLCO) 3.9 mmol/min/kPa
  (predicted 7.3–10.9)
Transfer coefficient for carbon monoxide (KCO)
  0.91 mmol/min/kPa/l (predicted 1.2–1.8)

Questions:

1. What type of defect is demonstrated by the changes in lung function?
2. What pathological process is likely to account for the findings in this patient?
3. Give two conditions which could account for the clinical picture in this patient.

Answers overleaf

11. 1. Chronic airflow limitation (chronic obstructive airways disease). The reduction in $FEV_1/FVC\%$ indicates airflow limitation, and the accompanying fall in gas transfer suggests that emphysema is an important contributing factor in this patient. The high haemoglobin value is probably the result of arterial hypoxaemia.

12. 1. A restrictive defect. The low KCO suggests the presence of lung parenchymal pathology (rather than a defect in the pleura, muscles of respiration, or chest wall).

2. Interstitial pulmonary fibrosis would account for the clubbing, radiological changes, restrictive defect, and low KCO.

3. Cryptogenic fibrosing alveolitis, connective tissue disorders such as scleroderma or systemic lupus erythematosus, and asbestosis are the diagnoses most likely to fit this picture. Extrinsic allergic alveolitis should be considered but it affects predominantly the upper zones on the chest radiograph, while sarcoidosis affects predominantly the mid zones and rarely causes clubbing.

13. A 68 year old man who has had back pain for many years, is found to have an early diastolic murmur. Chest radiograph shows bilateral apical shadowing but no evidence of heart failure.

Investigations showed:

FEV$_1$ 1.9 l (predicted 2.1–3.1)
FVC   2.4 l (predicted 3.0–4.4)
FEV$_1$/FVC   79%
Total lung capacity (TLC) 4.7 l (predicted 4.9–7.4)

Questions:

1. What type of defect is demonstrated by the changes in lung function?

2. What is the probable diagnosis?

14. A 55 year old previously healthy man who has never smoked develops a febrile illness with cough productive of yellow sputum accompanied by nausea, vomiting, and confusion. Chest radiograph shows shadowing in both lower zones.

Investigations showed:

Plasma sodium   124 mmol/l
       potassium   4.2 mmol/l
       urea   11.0 mmol/l
Serum creatinine   180 μmol/l
      bilirubin   23 μmol/l
      glutamic-oxaloacetic transaminase (GOT) 55 iu/l
      alkaline phosphatase   130 iu/l
Sputum: no growth on culture for bacteria.

Questions:

1. Give two likely diagnoses.

2. What treatment should be given?

Answers overleaf
79

13. 1. A restrictive defect is indicated by the low TLC, and high FEV_1/ FVC ratio.

   2. Ankylosing spondylitis, which is sometimes associated with aortic regurgitation, and with bilateral apical pulmonary shadowing, and a restrictive defect.

14. 1. The clinical picture of pneumonia with gastrointestinal symptoms, confusion, abnormal liver and renal function, and low plasma sodium raises the possibility of infection by *Legionella pneumophila*. Infection with *Mycoplasma pneumoniae* may cause similar abnormalities. Neither organism will be cultured from the sputum by routine bacteriological techniques.

   2. Both of these infections respond to treatment with erythromycin. Rifampicin is also effective against *L. pneumophila* and tetracycline against *M. pneumoniae*.

15. A 26 year old Nigerian man presents with night sweats. Chest radiograph shows bilateral hilar and mediastinal lymph node enlargement. General examination reveals no abnormality.

Investigations showed:

Hb   12.6 g/dl
WBC   7.3 x 10^9/l
ESR   55 mm in the first hour

Questions:

1. Give three possible diagnoses.

2. Give five further tests likely to establish the diagnosis.

16. A 50 year old non-smoking man works soldering components in an electronics factory. He develops an unproductive cough which is worse at night.

Investigations showed:

FEV_1 2.4 l (predicted 3.0–4.5)
FVC   3.8 l (predicted 3.9–5.9)
FEV_1/FVC   63%
Methacholine provocation test: concentration producing 20%
    fall in FEV_1 = 1 mg/ml (normal >4 mg/ml).

Questions:

1. What diagnosis is indicated by the tests of lung function?

2. What might have caused this disorder?

Answers overleaf

15. 1. Lymph node tuberculosis, sarcoidosis, and lymphoma can produce this appearance on chest radiograph and are the most likely diagnoses in this man.

2. Fibreoptic bronchoscopy and transbronchial biopsy might show evidence of pulmonary involvement in lymphoma or TB, and will reveal non-caseating granulomata in 80% of cases of sarcoidosis even in the absence of abnormality in the lung fields on chest radiograph. Tuberculin skin testing might be helpful since it is likely to be positive in tuberculosis but negative in sarcoidosis. If the diagnosis remains unclear, mediastinoscopy and lymph node biopsy are indicated.

The serum angiotensin converting enzyme may be elevated and Kveim test positive in sarcoidosis, but the delay inherent in obtaining the latter is unacceptable in this patient.

16. 1. The reduced FEV_1/FVC ratio (usually >70%) suggests the presence of airflow limitation. The methacholine provocation test indicates the presence of airway hyperresponsiveness. Taken together, these results suggest a diagnosis of asthma.

2. An occupational cause should be considered; solderers are at risk of developing occupational asthma which can be caused by fumes emitted from colophony resin in the solder wire, or by isocyanates liberated from polyurethane coating on the wire.

17. A 53 year old woman with seropositive rheumatoid arthritis develops gradually increasing breathlessness with finger clubbing and basal crackles. Chest radiograph shows bilateral basal shadowing.

Investigations showed:

FEV$_1$ 1.7 (predicted 1.8–2.8)
FVC   2.2 l (predicted 2.4–3.6)
FEV$_1$/FVC   77%
Total lung capacity (TLC) 3.6 l (predicted 3.8–5.7)
Transfer coefficient for carbon monoxide 1.1 mmol/min/kPa/l
    (predicted 1.4–2.0)

Questions:

1. What is the most likely cause of her breathlessness?

2. How would you confirm this diagnosis?

18. A 22 year old woman presents with a two hour history of breathlessness. There is tachypnoea but examination is otherwise normal, and chest radiograph is normal.

Investigations showed:

Arterial blood (breathing air):
    PO$_2$ 12.2 kPa (92 mm Hg)
    PCO$_2$ 3.2 kPa (24 mm Hg)
    pH   7.54
    Bicarbonate   20 mmol/l

Hb   13.5 g/dl

Questions:

1. What abnormality is demonstrated by the arterial blood gas results?

2. What is the probable cause in this patient and what would be your management?

Answers overleaf

17. 1. Fibrosing alveolitis is associated with rheumatoid arthritis, and would account for the restrictive defect, clubbing, basal crackles, and radiological findings. Patients with rheumatoid arthritis also have an increased incidence of bronchiectasis, which can also cause clubbing and basal crackles. The history is not suggestive of bronchiectasis however, and the lung function tests often show airflow limitation in this condition.

2. Fibreoptic bronchoscopy and transbronchial biopsy may allow a histological diagnosis of fibrosing alveolitis but if negative, confirmation of this diagnosis will require an open lung biopsy. In practice, many patients may be successfully managed without histological confirmation of the diagnosis.

18. 1. Respiratory alkalosis; the elevated pH indicates the presence of alkalosis, and the low $PaCO_2$ indicates that there is hyperventilation.

2. The abnormality is very likely to be caused by anxiety since there is no evidence of a respiratory or metabolic stimulus to hyperventilation. The possibility of pulmonary emboli must however be considered in this patient and if there is doubt an isotope lung scan should be done. Patients with hyperventilation related to anxiety require reassurance, and if symptoms of tetany develop, rebreathing from a bag may be helpful by bringing about an increase in the $PaCO_2$. Investigation and appropriate management of underlying stress and psychological problems is necessary if recurrent attacks occur.

19. A 50 year old man with longstanding asthma and productive cough develops a fever, with increased wheeze and sputum production. Chest radiograph shows bilateral upper zone shadowing which was not present on his last chest radiograph taken five years previously. Investigations showed:

Hb   13.6 g/dl
WBC   8.9 x 10^9/l, 60% neutrophils,12% eosinophils, 20% lymphocytes,8% monocytes
ESR   65 mm in the first hour
Sputum negative for acid alcohol fast bacilli (AAFB) (three samples)

Questions:

1. List two likely causes of the radiological changes.

2. List five investigations to determine the cause.

20. A 73 year old man is admitted to hospital with an infective exacerbation of chronic airflow limitation. Investigations showed:

Arterial blood (breathing air):

PO_2 6.5 kPa (49 mm Hg)
PCO_2 7.1 kPa (53 mm Hg)
pH   7.31
Bicarbonate 26 mmol/l

He is treated with 24% oxygen. Two hours later he is drowsy and arterial blood gases show:

PO_2 9.8 kPa (74 mm Hg)
PCO_2 9.3 kPa (70 mm Hg)
pH   7.23
Bicarbonate 28 mmol/l

Questions:

1. What is the probable reason for his drowsiness?

2. What treatment does he require to correct this complication?

Answers overleaf

19. 1. Pulmonary tuberculosis must be excluded, in spite of the absence of AAFB in the sputum. Allergic bronchopulmonary aspergillosis (ABPA) should also be considered in view of the eosinophilia, history of asthma, chronic sputum production, and upper zone shadowing on chest radiograph. The distribution of radiological changes makes other causes of bronchopulmonary eosinophilia less likely.

2. Fibreoptic bronchoscopy with bronchial lavage and trans-bronchial biopsy may demonstrate AAFB and/or caseating granulomata in tuberculosis. A diagnosis of ABPA would be supported by a positive skin prick test and the presence of serum precipitins to *Aspergillus fumigatus*. Additional tests include estimation of serum IgE levels to *Aspergillus fumigatus*, and the organism may be found in the sputum or bronchial aspirate.

20. 1. Carbon dioxide retention secondary to hypoventilation. In patients with chronic airflow limitation and hypercapnia, toler-ance develops to the respiratory stimulant effects of carbon dioxide. As a result, hypoxaemia becomes a more important stimulus to ventilation. In such patients the diminution of hypoxaemia following oxygen therapy causes a reduction in ventilation and consequent increase in $PaCO_2$.

2. Usually, treatment with 24% oxygen is uncomplicated but some patients cannot tolerate even this, as in the present case. Use of a respiratory stimulant such as intravenous doxapram infusion may be sufficient to allow correction of the underlying causes of the patient's deterioration. However, it may become necessary to consider positive pressure ventilation.

INDEX

A LATE HARVEST